Women with ADHD

Healthy Mind

Olivia I. Thigpen ENG

Published by Digital Mind, 2023.

WOMEN WITH ADHD

First edition. December 18, 2023.

ISBN: 979-8215736579

Written by Olivia I. Thigpen ENG.

Also by Olivia I. Thigpen ENG

Healthy Mind
The Overthinking Cure: 8 Proven Strategies to Free Your Mind from Negative Spirals, Reduce Stress, Boost Productivity, and Live in the Present Moment
Love amidst Anxiety: How to Build Healthy Relationships in Uncertain Times
Women with ADHD

Healthy Relationships
Breaking Free from Narcissistic Manipulation: Strategies for Healing and Thriving Beyond Toxic Relationships
Narcissistic Relationships: Overcoming Codependency, Setting Boundaries, and Healing Romantic Bonds in a Turbulent World

Table of Contents

Introduction

In the complex tapestry of human diversity, attention and hyperactivity play crucial roles in how we experience and navigate the world. Over the years, Attention Deficit Hyperactivity Disorder (ADHD) has been a constantly evolving area of research and understanding. However, in this exploration, one specific facet has often been underestimated or overlooked: the impact of ADHD on women.

This book is a work that seeks to fill that void, offering a deep and comprehensive look at the unique experience of women living with ADHD. Through these pages, we will embark on a journey of discovery, empowerment and transformation, exploring the complexities of this disorder from a perspective that has historically been less visible.

To fully understand the narrative of women with ADHD, it is crucial to place this disorder in its broader context. ADHD, characterized by difficulty maintaining attention, impulsivity and hyperactivity, has been studied mainly from childhood to adolescence. However, in women, these manifestations can present differently and often go unnoticed. Stigma and lack of awareness have contributed to many women living with ADHD without proper diagnosis or treatment.

Women with ADHD face a unique set of challenges in their daily lives. From organizing time to managing interpersonal relationships, every aspect of life can be influenced by the interaction of ADHD in women. This book sets out to address these challenges head-on, providing specific strategies and tools designed to empower women to overcome distractions, improve their relationships, and find success in multiple facets of life.

The path to understanding and managing ADHD in women begins with an accurate diagnosis. However, the complexity of symptoms in women often leads to misdiagnosis or lack of recognition. We will thoroughly explore the diagnosis and evaluation process, highlighting common challenges and offering valuable information on specialized tools and tests that can improve diagnostic accuracy.

One of the most pressing challenges women with ADHD face is organizing their time. This book will provide practical strategies to develop effective organizational skills, create personalized routines, and leverage technological tools that facilitate time management, thus allowing women to maximize their productivity and achieve their daily goals.

Everyday distractions can become significant obstacles for women with ADHD. We'll explore common distractions, from the most obvious to the most subtle, and provide effective techniques for maintaining focus. Additionally, we will examine how to create environments conducive to concentration, both at home and at work.

ADHD can have a significant impact on personal relationships. We will address how women with ADHD can communicate effectively with friends and family, build healthy relationships, and overcome interpersonal challenges.

Throughout this journey, we will delve into the complexity of emotions, explore strategies for emotional management, and examine the impact of ADHD on women's mental health and emotional well-being. From financial management to career development, this book will be a comprehensive guide that addresses every aspect of the life of a woman with ADHD.

This book seeks to inspire, empower, and provide the tools necessary for women to succeed in life, regardless of the challenges that ADHD may present. With a mix of up-to-date research, personal experiences, and practical advice, this book serves as a compass for women seeking to successfully navigate the waters of life with ADHD.

Chapter 1: Understanding ADHD in Women

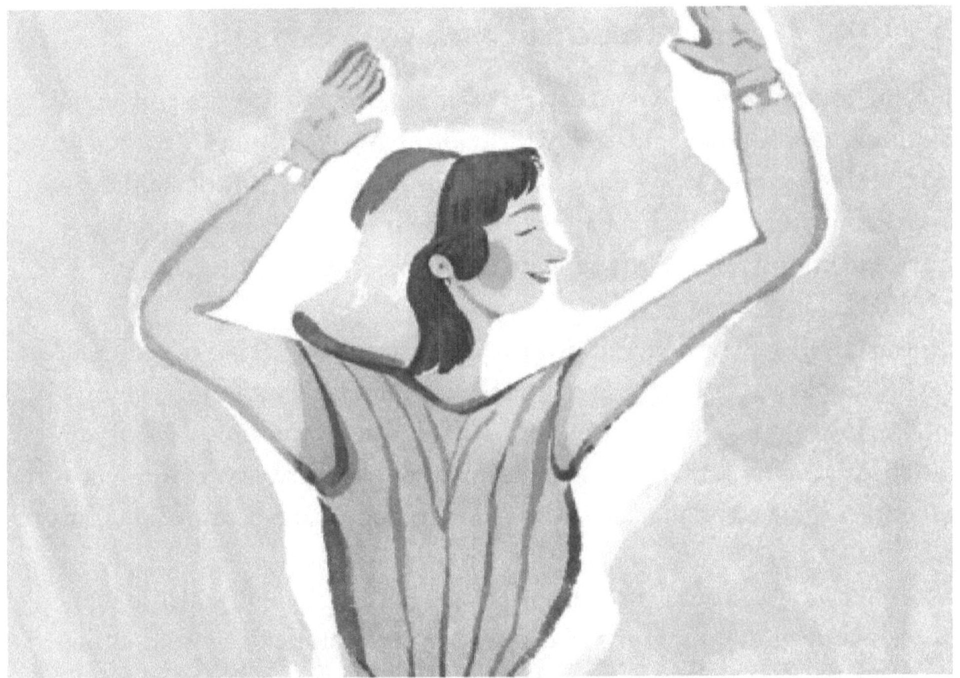

Over the decades, ADHD has been the subject of extensive study, yet women's unique experience with this disorder has often been overshadowed by the mainstream narrative.

This first chapter seeks to illuminate that dark corner and offer a detailed look at ADHD in women. Beyond the conventional image of ADHD, we will explore the specific complexities that women face when living with this disorder. From childhood to adulthood, understanding how ADHD manifests in women is essential to providing appropriate and personalized support.

Through a comprehensive approach, this chapter aims to distill the essence of ADHD, shedding light on its nuances in the female context. From the challenges it poses to the unique strengths it can bring, we will explore every facet of this disorder to build a solid foundation that allows women to not only understand it but also approach it with resilience and determination.

Understanding ADHD in women goes beyond a simple description of symptoms; It involves immersing yourself in individual experiences, recognizing patterns, and most importantly, challenging ingrained stereotypes that have perpetuated misunderstandings about how this disorder manifests in women.

1.1 Introduction to ADHD

Imagine your mind as a river, constantly flowing, sometimes calm and serene, and at other times, full of rapids and whirlpools. Now, imagine this river is in your head, and sometimes those rapids and eddies can make it a little harder to focus on one thing for very long. That's what happens in some people's minds, and we call it Attention Deficit Hyperactivity Disorder, or ADHD.

<u>ADHD in Simple Words</u>

ADHD is like having a mind that jumps from one thing to another like a playful monkey in a jungle. Sometimes it is difficult to stay focused on a task because the mind is excited by many different ideas at the same time. But it's not just about attention, there is also an element of hyperactivity, which means that sometimes there is too much energy, as if your body wants to move and can't stay still!

Think of it as having a superpower of super energy and super imagination, but sometimes, this superpower can also make it difficult to follow the rules or stay in one place for too long. It's not that you don't want to do it, it's just that your mind and body are so excited that they want to explore and discover everything at once.

<u>The Differences Between Boys and Girls with ADHD</u>

Before, many people thought that only children had ADHD, but that is not true! Girls can have it too, it just sometimes manifests itself a little differently. While in boys hyperactivity may be more obvious, in girls hyperactivity may be expressed more internally, as if they have a whirlwind of ideas spinning in their heads!

Plus, girls with ADHD are often very good at hiding it. They may try hard to appear as if they are paying attention and being orderly, but inside, their mental river is still flowing rapidly. This can sometimes make it harder for girls to get help because it is not always easy to see.

How ADHD is Diagnosed

Diagnosing ADHD is not like solving a simple puzzle. There is no single test that can tell for sure if someone has ADHD. Instead, doctors and health professionals look at many aspects of a person's life, how they behave, how they concentrate, and how they manage their energy. They also ask parents, teachers and sometimes the person themselves about their daily life.

The diagnosis process is like putting together a puzzle with many different pieces: observations, questions, and personal experiences. Only when all the pieces fit together can you say for sure if someone has ADHD.

The Superpower of ADHD and the Challenges It Brings

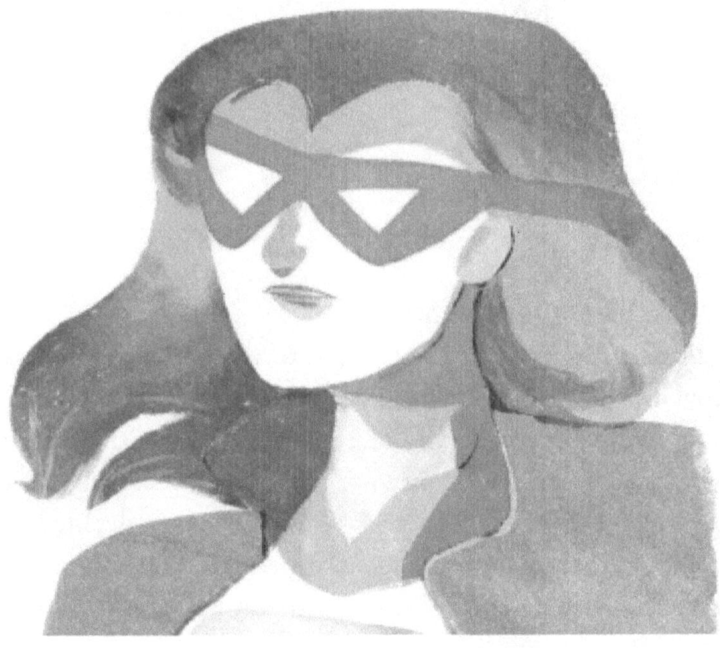

Having ADHD is not just a set of challenges; It also comes with some amazing superpowers . Imagine having the ability to think about many things at once, be creative, and have unlimited energy when you are truly passionate about something. These are the positive sides of ADHD that often go unnoticed.

However, with superpowers also come challenges. It can be difficult to focus on a task for a long time, follow rules, or remember important little things.

Sometimes this can make people with ADHD feel bad about themselves or wonder why they can't be like everyone else.

1.2 Gender differences in ADHD

1. Why Do Gender Differences Matter?

First, let's talk about why it's important to explore the differences between girls and boys with ADHD. Before, many people thought that only boys had ADHD, but now we know that girls have it too. The thing is, sometimes ADHD in girls can be like a wizard hiding in a hat, sometimes it's not so easy to see!

Recognizing these differences is like having a more detailed map on our journey. It helps us better understand how girls and boys uniquely experience and cope with the challenges of ADHD, which is key to providing appropriate support.

2. The Tides of ADHD in Boys and Girls

Imagine ADHD as waves in an ocean. In boys, these waves may be higher and more visible, like when you are playing on a beach and the waves hit you hard. But on girls, the waves can be more subtle, like when you're standing on a calm shore and the waves gently wash at your feet.

In boys, hyperactivity is often like those big waves. They can be very active, move a lot and be noticeable in their energy. In girls, hyperactivity can be more internal, as if they have a hurricane of ideas spinning in their minds. Although it's not always visible from the outside, it can be just as powerful!

3. The Art of Hiding ADHD

Girls with ADHD are sometimes like artists who hide their art. They may try hard to appear like they are paying attention and being organized, but inside, their mental river is still flowing rapidly. This sometimes makes it harder for the girls to get help, like they're wearing a magic cloak that hides their superpower !

This art of hiding ADHD can lead to misunderstandings. Girls may feel like they have to be perfect to fit the mold that society expects of them. But here's an important secret: no one is perfect! We all have our own unique ways of shining, and ADHD is just part of what makes us special.

4. Differences in Diagnosis: Personalized Puzzles

Diagnosing ADHD in girls can be like solving a personalized puzzle. There is no one piece that fits all. Health professionals look at many different things, such as behavior, attention, and energy, to put the puzzle together. They talk to parents, teachers, and sometimes even the girls themselves to understand what their daily lives are like.

This process is like designing a puzzle that fits perfectly into each person's unique life. It's a reminder that we are all different and unique, and that is a beautiful thing.

5. The Hidden Strength: Female Superpowers with ADHD

Despite the challenges, girls with ADHD also have hidden superpowers . Imagine having the ability to think about many things at once, be creative, and have unlimited energy when you are truly passionate about something. These are amazing superpowers that are often overlooked.

The creativity of girls with ADHD can be like a secret garden full of bright, shiny flowers. Sometimes these flowers can be distractions, but they can also be incredible ideas that blossom into something wonderful.

6. How to Help Girls with ADHD Shine

Now that we've explored these differences, the question is: how can we help girls with ADHD shine even brighter? A key part is recognizing and celebrating your unique superpowers . Allowing them to be themselves and supporting their talents can open avenues for them to explore and grow.

It is also crucial to provide an environment where they can feel comfortable sharing their challenges. Instead of hiding behind the magic cloak, let's encourage them to talk openly and honestly about their experiences. In doing so, we are building bridges of understanding and support.

In short, exploring gender differences in ADHD is like discovering hidden treasure. By understanding how the mental river flows uniquely in girls, we can build stronger bridges, provide more effective support, and create a journey that celebrates both the challenges and superpowers of each person.

1.3 Specific challenges for women with ADHD

The Dance of Challenges in the Feminine Mental River

ADHD in women often presents unique challenges, like a special dance in the mental river. While some girls may have a more serene river, others may feel that their waters are full of unexpected twists and turns. These challenges can affect different areas of daily life, from organization to relationships and beyond.

Challenge number one: The Battle for Organization

One of the areas where women with ADHD may encounter significant challenges is in organization. Keeping everything in its place can feel like trying to catch butterflies in a garden full of flowers. Although some women may have innate organizational skills, others may struggle with the task of putting all the pieces in place.

This challenge does not mean that women with ADHD are not able to organize, but rather that they may need specific strategies and additional support to do so effectively!

Challenge number two: The Game of Interpersonal Relationships

Personal relationships can also be like a complicated game for women with ADHD. The dance in their minds can sometimes make it difficult to follow conversations or remember important details. This doesn't mean they don't value their relationships, but sometimes they need a little more understanding and patience from others.

The challenge here is to find ways to communicate effectively, express your needs, and maintain healthy relationships. It's like learning a new dance, where every step counts and the emotional connection becomes a masterpiece.

Challenge number three: The Labyrinth of Emotions

ADHD in women can also affect emotional management. Emotions can be like an ever-changing maze, where finding the right path can be a challenge. Sometimes these emotions can be intense and difficult to understand, adding an extra layer of complexity to everyday life.

This challenge does not mean that women with ADHD are emotionally unstable, but rather that they may need specific strategies to recognize, understand, and regulate their emotions in healthy ways.

Challenge Number Four: Struggling with Social Expectations

Social expectations can also become a challenge for women with ADHD. There is often pressure to fit into certain molds and meet predefined standards. The unique dance of their minds can cause them to follow their own rhythm, sometimes divergent from external expectations.

This challenge does not mean that women with ADHD cannot meet expectations, but rather that they may need flexibility and understanding in the process. The key is to allow each woman to define her own success and path in life.

Overcoming Challenges with Specific Strategies

Although these challenges may seem like towering mountains, it is important to remember that each challenge is also an opportunity to grow and learn. Through specific strategies, women with ADHD can overcome these obstacles and thrive in their lives.

Organization can be improved with personalized routines and the help of technological tools. Relationships can be strengthened through open communication and building meaningful connections. Emotional management can improve with well-being practices and the search for balance. When it comes to social expectations, the key is to embrace authenticity and challenge restrictive standards.

Chapter 2: Diagnosis and Evaluation in Women

On our journey toward understanding and empowering women with Attention Deficit Hyperactivity Disorder (ADHD), we delve into a crucial chapter: the diagnosis and evaluation process. This leg of the journey is like a thorough exploration, where we unravel the specific complexities surrounding identifying and understanding ADHD in women.

Understanding how the diagnosis is carried out is essential. It is not simply a stamp that is placed on a sheet of paper, but a delicate and personalized process that seeks to put together a unique puzzle for each woman. In this chapter, we will explore the particularities of this process, the challenges it can present and how it can become a fundamental tool for empowerment and improving the quality of life.

2.1 Diagnostic process

A) The Personalized ADHD Puzzle

Diagnosing ADHD is not like a one-time yes or no test. It's more like putting together a puzzle. Every woman has a unique puzzle , with pieces that include her behavior, her way of thinking, and how she interacts with the world around her. The diagnostic process is the task of putting all of these pieces together and seeing how they fit together.

B) Important Observations: The Dance of Warning Signs

The first step in the diagnostic process often involves careful observation. Health professionals, such as doctors and psychologists, look for warning signs that could indicate the presence of ADHD. These signals can manifest in different ways compared to men, as the dance of female minds is sometimes more subtle.

Patterns can be seen in the way a woman pays attention, organizes her time, or manages emotions. Are you easily distracted? Do you have difficulty concentrating on a task? These are some of the clues that could lead to a deeper understanding.

C) Interviews and Talks: Deciphering Personal History

After the observations, comes the stage of interviews and talks. Here, the health professional can speak directly with the woman, and sometimes with her family members or teachers, to obtain a more complete view of her personal history. Questions about childhood, school life and relationships can help you unravel the puzzle .

It's like telling the story of a life: what was it like growing up, facing challenges, and learning to deal with the world? These conversations are crucial to understanding each woman's unique experience with ADHD.

D) Special Tools: Tests and Evaluations

In addition to observations and conversations, special tools are used to obtain more detailed information. These tools may include tests and assessments designed specifically to evaluate ADHD. These tests can measure attention, impulsivity, and hyperactivity, thus providing more objective data on mental and emotional functioning.

Imagine these tests as special lenses that help focus the image. They provide key information that can be essential in reaching a clear and accurate diagnosis.

E) Coexisting Conditions: Unmasking Other Challenges

ADHD sometimes travels accompanied by other conditions. It's as if the detective discovers that there is more than one story at play. It is common for women with ADHD to also experience anxiety, depression, or other mental health conditions. The diagnostic process also seeks to identify these co-occurring conditions to ensure a comprehensive approach to healthcare.

F) Unique Challenges in Female Diagnosis

Diagnosing ADHD in women presents unique challenges. Sometimes the characteristics of ADHD can be more difficult to recognize due to the coping strategies that women have developed. They may have learned to hide certain behaviors or compensate effectively, which can make red flags less obvious.

Additionally, lack of awareness about ADHD in women can lead to misunderstandings and misdiagnoses. That is why this diagnostic process is so essential; seeks to go beyond appearances and explore the unique reality of each woman.

2.2 Common obstacles in diagnosis in women

Obstacle number one: Stereotypes and Social Expectations

One of the biggest obstacles in diagnosing ADHD in women lies in ingrained stereotypes and social expectations. The traditional idea of a person with ADHD often centers on the image of a hyperactive and distracted child. This stereotype can obscure understanding of how ADHD manifests in women, as their experience may be less visible and more internal.

Social expectations also play a crucial role. Women are expected to be organized, attentive and able to handle multiple tasks without problems. When these expectations clash with characteristics of ADHD, such as difficulty maintaining attention or organization, misunderstandings and obstacles can arise on the path to diagnosis.

Obstacle number two : Efficient Coping Strategies

Women with ADHD often develop very efficient coping strategies to deal with the challenges they face. These strategies may include a conscious effort to appear organized, pay attention, and meet social expectations. Although these strategies are valuable and reflect the resilience of women with ADHD, they can also act as veils that hide underlying symptoms.

This camouflage can make it difficult for healthcare professionals and those around you to easily spot the warning signs of ADHD. The woman may be so accustomed to compensating for her challenges that she may not even recognize the need for help.

Obstacle number three: Lack of Awareness and Education

Lack of awareness and education about ADHD in women is another major obstacle. Sometimes, neither women nor those around them are familiar with the variety of ways ADHD can manifest in the female gender. This can lead to lack of recognition of symptoms and therefore a delay in diagnosis.

Education is a powerful tool to overcome this obstacle. Increasing awareness of how ADHD manifests in women, promoting understanding of individual variations, and eliminating stereotypes contributes to creating an environment in which diagnosis can be more accurate and timely.

Obstacle number four: Traditional Non-Adapted Assessments

Traditional assessments used to diagnose ADHD are often based on models designed to detect the disorder in children, and these are not always adapted for gender differences. Women with ADHD may not easily fit established criteria, as their symptoms may be less evident or manifest differently.

Tailoring assessments to include specific aspects of how ADHD presents in women is essential. This involves considering not only external hyperactivity but also internal hyperactivity, inattention, and other nuances that may be more subtle.

Obstacle Number Five: Coexisting Diagnosis of Other Mental Health Conditions

ADHD is often accompanied by other mental health conditions, such as anxiety or depression. The presence of these conditions can complicate diagnosis, as symptoms can overlap or mask each other. Identifying ADHD specifically among other conditions may require careful analysis and a deep understanding of the interaction between different aspects of mental health.

Overcoming Obstacles to Accurate Diagnosis

Although these obstacles may seem challenging, it is important to remember that overcoming them is possible. The key is to address each obstacle with specific, personalized approaches. Consciousness, both at the individual level and at the societal level , plays a crucial role in this process. Education, adapting assessments, and understanding coping strategies are essential tools to overcome these obstacles and achieve a more accurate diagnosis.

2.3 Specialized tools and tests for women with ADHD

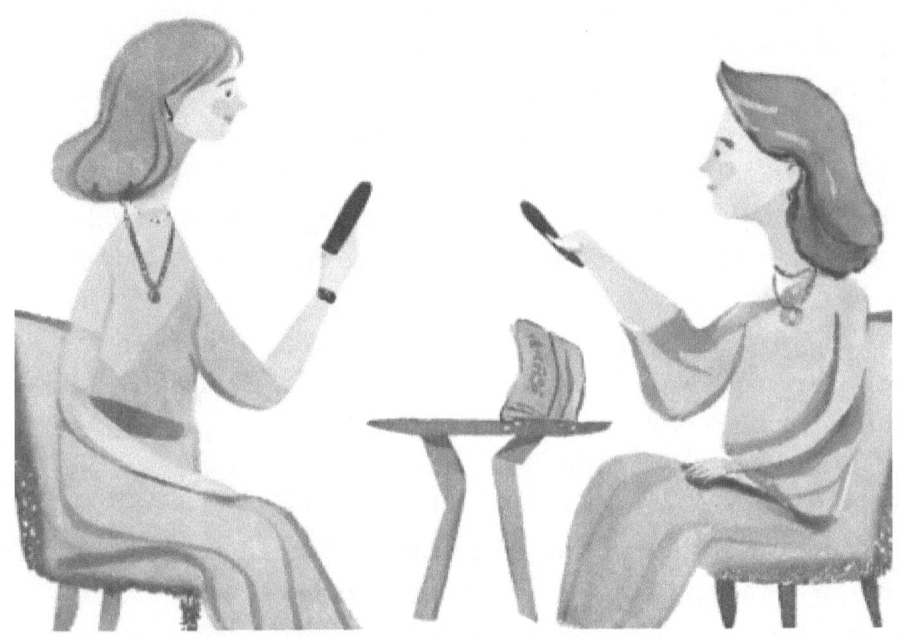

1. Detailed Interviews: Unraveling Personal Stories

In-depth interviews are like deep conversations that seek to unravel the personal stories of women with ADHD. Here, health professionals speak directly to women and sometimes to their family members or teachers. Questions about childhood, daily life, and relationships provide valuable clues about how ADHD manifests in everyday life.

These interviews not only gather information about overt symptoms, but also explore coping strategies that women may have developed. By analyzing these strategies, professionals can gain a more complete view of each woman's unique experience with ADHD.

2. Scales and Specific Questionnaires for Women

Specialized scales and questionnaires are tools designed specifically to assess ADHD in women. Unlike more general tests, these tools take into account gender differences in the presentation of ADHD symptoms. Tailored questions can address internal hyperactivity, inattention, and other issues that may be more subtle in women.

These tools are like maps designed specifically to navigate the waters of female ADHD. They provide a framework that helps professionals identify patterns and more accurately assess the presence and severity of the disorder.

3. Evaluation of Coping Strategies

Women with ADHD often develop ingenious strategies to deal with daily challenges. These strategies may include to-do lists, visual reminders, or specific methods for staying focused. Analyzing these strategies not only reveals women's creativity and resilience , but also provides clues to the underlying challenges they face.

Assessing coping strategies is like cracking a code. It helps to understand how women with ADHD have learned to manage their challenges and what additional supports may be beneficial in their daily lives.

4. Evaluation of Coexisting Conditions

ADHD is often accompanied by other mental health conditions, such as anxiety or depression. Evaluating these coexisting conditions is like exploring additional terrain on our journey. Health professionals look at how these conditions interact with each other and how they affect a woman's overall life.

Identifying and addressing these co-occurring conditions is critical to providing comprehensive treatment. It's like treating not only the symptoms of ADHD, but also understanding how other conditions can influence a woman's overall experience.

5. Evaluation of the Executive Function

The executive function is like the director of a play. Controls the mental and cognitive skills necessary to carry out tasks and goals. In women with ADHD, executive function may be impaired, which may manifest in difficulties planning, organizing, and completing tasks.

Executive function assessments are specialized tools that help measure these skills. They examine how a woman approaches daily tasks, how she organizes herself, and how she plans her time. These assessments are like flashlights that illuminate specific areas that may need additional support.

6. Benefits of Specialized Tools

Using specialized tools and tests in the diagnosis of ADHD in women offers significant benefits. These tools not only allow for a more precise and detailed assessment, but also recognize and assess gender differences in the presentation of ADHD. Additionally, tailoring assessments overcomes obstacles that could arise due to stereotypes or pre-existing expectations.

By employing these tools, the diagnostic process becomes a thorough exploration, guided by an understanding of the individual experiences of women with ADHD. This targeted, personalized approach not only improves diagnostic accuracy, but also lays the foundation for tailored strategies and supports that will make a difference in daily life.

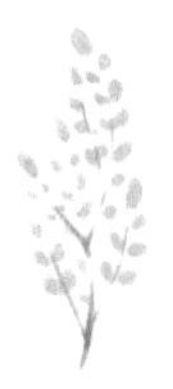

Chapter 3: Organization and Time Management Strategies

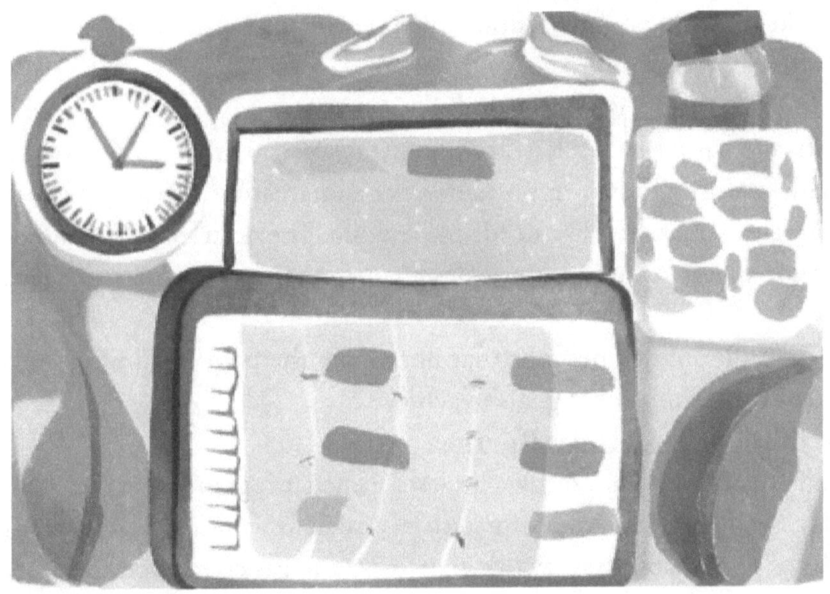

In our journey through the journey of women with Attention Deficit Hyperactivity Disorder (ADHD), we reach crucial ground: the development of organizational skills. This section is like a practical workshop where we will explore tools and strategies that will help women build solid foundations for the organization in their daily lives. So, let's get to work and explore how developing organizational skills can be a valuable compass on the path to a more structured and fulfilling life.

3.1 Development of organizational skills

<u>Understanding Organizational Skills</u>

Imagine organizational skills as an artist's tools before starting a masterpiece. They are essential for structuring and shaping daily life. In the context of ADHD, these skills become even more critical as they help mitigate the challenges associated with distraction and inattention.

Creating Organized Spaces

The first step in developing organizational skills is creating orderly spaces. This means setting up specific areas for tasks and objects, such as a desk for work or a designated place for keys. Keeping these spaces organized helps reduce the chance of distractions and makes it easier to locate important items when they are needed.

It's like drawing boundaries on a map; Each area has its purpose and is kept orderly for easy navigation.

Using Lists and Visual Reminders

Lists and visual reminders are like detailed maps that guide you through daily tasks. Writing down important tasks and creating visual reminders helps you keep clear track of what needs to be done. They can be simple notes stuck in strategic places or applications designed for visual reminders on electronic devices.

These tools are like beacons that illuminate the path, reminding women of what steps to take and what goals to achieve.

Establishing Consistent Routines

Consistent routines are like pre-established programs that help structure your day. Setting specific times for activities such as working, eating, and resting provides a predictable framework that makes it easier to focus and organize. Additionally, routines provide a sense of order and stability.

It's like following a familiar route; Women with ADHD can anticipate what's next, making it easier to transition between activities.

Prioritizing Tasks Effectively

Effective task prioritization is like choosing the best routes on a map. It is essential to identify the most important and urgent tasks to tackle them first. This prevents women from feeling overwhelmed and allows them to focus their energy on what really matters.

By prioritizing, a clear path is established that guides towards meeting goals and objectives.

Leveraging Organizational Technologies

Organizational technologies are like virtual personal assistants. Apps and online tools can be powerful allies for women with ADHD. Electronic calendars, to-do list apps, and automatic reminders are valuable resources that can be easily integrated into everyday life.

These technologies act as electronic guides, keeping women on the right course and ensuring that no important task is left behind.

Learning to Delegate Responsibilities

Learning to delegate responsibilities is like sharing the burden of the journey. It is not necessary to tackle all tasks alone. Delegating means asking for help when necessary and distributing responsibilities among family, friends or colleagues. This relieves the burden and allows you to focus on what is most important. It's like having travel companions who share the journey, making the trip more bearable.

Benefits of Developing Organizational Skills

Developing organizational skills not only makes daily life easier, but also offers significant benefits for women with ADHD. By creating structure and routines, you reduce the stress and anxiety associated with a lack of organization. Additionally, these skills provide a solid framework for success in various areas, from work to personal relationships. Developing organizational skills is a powerful ally on the journey toward a more structured and satisfying life.

3.2 Creating effective routines

Understanding the Importance of Routines

Routines are like maps that trace a predictable path through the daily hustle and bustle. For women with ADHD, establishing effective routines can be a valuable tool to counteract the challenges of distraction and inattention. Let's see how these routines become essential allies on the journey towards organization and well-being.

1. Establishing Consistent Schedules

Imagine the schedule as the skeleton that shapes the day. Setting consistent schedules for key activities, such as waking up, working, and resting, provides a solid framework. This not only helps maintain structure, but also makes it easier to transition between different tasks.

It's like following a script; Women can anticipate what's next, which reduces uncertainty and promotes concentration.

2. Including Time for Rest and Recovery

Including moments to rest and recover is like adding rest areas along the way. Women with ADHD can easily feel overwhelmed, and taking time to recharge is crucial. These rest periods not only improve emotional well-being, but also contribute to more sustainable performance over time.

It's like planning rest areas on a long trip; It allows you to enjoy the landscape without getting exhausted.

3. Customizing Routines according to Individual Preferences

Every woman is unique, and her routines should reflect those uniquenesses. Customizing routines based on individual preferences is like designing a custom trip. Some women may prefer to work in the morning, while others are more productive in the afternoon. Respecting these preferences contributes to greater efficiency and satisfaction.

It's like adapting a trip itinerary to personal interests and needs; It becomes more meaningful and enjoyable.

4. Incorporating Pleasurable Activities

Incorporating pleasurable activities into your routine is like adding exciting destinations to your trip. Women with ADHD may benefit from including time for activities they enjoy, whether it's reading, exercising, or pursuing creative hobbies. These moments not only bring joy but also act as a positive pick-me-up amidst daily responsibilities.

It's like planning stops on a trip to enjoy experiences that bring happiness and renewal.

5. Flexibility to Adapt to Changes

Flexibility in routines is like having an updated map during the trip. Life is full of unexpected events, and women with ADHD can face sudden changes. Maintaining flexibility allows you to adapt to new circumstances without feeling overwhelmed. Being able to adjust the routine as needed contributes to a feeling of control and adaptability.

It's like having a plan B on the trip; Alternative routes can be explored when necessary.

6. Using Visual Reminders and Alarms

Visual reminders and alarms are like signposts along the way. They can be useful tools for remembering important tasks or transitions between activities. These visual and auditory aids act as friendly guides that keep women on track, avoiding forgetfulness or distractions. It's like having a co-pilot who advises you about the next steps in the journey, ensuring that nothing is left behind.

Benefits of Effective Routines

Effective routines not only bring structure to daily life, but also offer significant benefits for women with ADHD. By providing an organized framework, routines reduce the stress and anxiety associated with a lack of structure. In addition, they contribute to better time management and more consistent performance in various areas. By building effective routines, women are not only designing their days, they are creating a framework for a more balanced and satisfying journey.

3.3 Use of technological tools for time management

Understanding the Importance of Technological Tools

Technological tools are like bright beacons in the daily commute. For women with ADHD, these tools can be powerful allies in addressing the challenges associated with distraction and inattention. Let's take a look at how these technological tools can be effectively integrated to improve time management.

A) Electronic Calendars: The Digital Agenda

Electronic calendars are like digital agendas that guide you through time. These tools allow you to schedule events, set reminders, and view the day clearly. They can sync with multiple devices, ensuring information is always within reach.

It's like having an interactive weather map; Women can plan and anticipate events, making preparation and organization easier.

B) To-Do List Apps: Reminders in Your Pocket

To-do list apps are like reminders in your pocket. They allow you to create detailed task lists, assign priorities, and check off items as they are completed. These applications are versatile and can adapt to different organizational styles.

It's like having a personal assistant who constantly keeps track of pending tasks, making sure nothing is left behind.

C) Automatic Reminders: Allies at the Opportune Moment

Automatic reminders are like friends that alert you at the right time. They can be set to remind you of specific tasks at designated times. These reminders can be visual, auditory or even tactile, adapting to individual preferences.

It's like receiving little signals throughout the day; It helps you stay on track and remember the essentials.

D) Personal Organization Apps: Everything in One Place

Personal organization apps are like virtual toolboxes. They can include calendar features, to-do lists, reminders, and more. These applications integrate various tools in one place, simplifying time management.

It's like having a digital command center; All the necessary tools are within reach, making organization easier.

E) Timers and Alarms: Setting the Rhythm

Timers and alarms are like digital hourglasses. They can be used to divide time into specific intervals and pace activities. These tools are particularly useful for avoiding procrastination and maintaining focus.

It's like having a training partner who marks the beginning and end of each task, encouraging discipline.

F) Time Tracking Apps: Knowing Where Time Goes

Time tracking apps are like mirrors that reflect how each minute is used. These applications record time spent on different activities, offering valuable information about time use patterns. This allows adjustments to be made to improve efficiency.

It's like keeping a detailed record of the trip; provides a clear view of how time is allocated and where improvements can be made.

How to Wisely Integrate Technological Tools

The key to getting the most out of technological tools is to integrate them wisely into your daily routine. Here are some practical tips:

- Select Adapted Tools: Choose tools that suit individual preferences and needs. Customization is key to a successful integration.
- Set Reminders to Use Tools: Setting regular reminders to review technology tools ensures they are used consistently.
- Learn and Upgrade: Spend time learning about the features and upgrades of your selected tools. Staying updated maximizes the benefit they can bring.
- Experiment with Different Apps: Not all apps are the same. Experimenting with different options allows you to find those that best fit specific needs.

- Integrate into the Daily Routine: Incorporating the use of technological tools into the daily routine is essential. They can become beneficial habits over time.

Benefits of Using Technological Tools for Time Management

Effectively incorporating technological tools in time management offers significant benefits. These tools act as facilitators, helping to overcome the challenges associated with ADHD. By providing reminders, organizing tasks, and visualizing time, women can experience a noticeable improvement in efficiency and a sense of control over their days.

Chapter 4: Overcoming Everyday Distractions

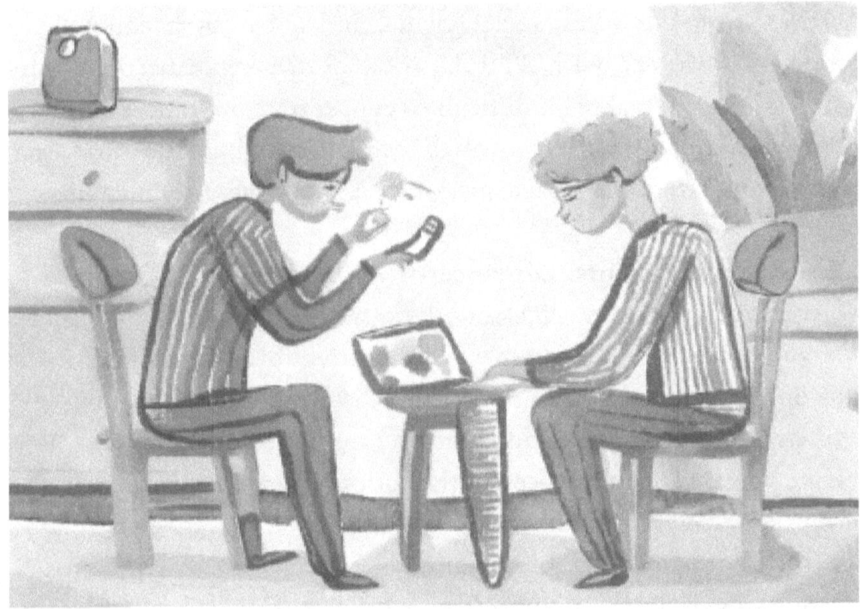

As we journey down the path of understanding and supporting women with Attention Deficit Hyperactivity Disorder (ADHD), we face a crucial challenge: identifying common distractions. These distractions are like traffic signs on our daily commute, and recognizing them is the first step to overcoming them. In this section, we will explore the distractions that often enter the scene, diverting us from our goals and committing ourselves to the task of overcoming them. Join us as we discover how identifying these distractions can be the key to clearing the path to greater focus and success.

4.1 Identification of common distractions

Understanding Everyday Distractions

Everyday distractions are like unexpected intruders on our journey. They can manifest in different ways and in different environments, affecting concentration and productivity. For women with ADHD, identifying these common distractions is essential to being able to address them effectively. Let's look at some of the distractions that frequently occur in daily life:

1. Electronic Devices: Digital Temptations

Electronic devices are like flashing beacons that capture our attention. Notifications from messages, social media, and apps can become significant distractions. For women with ADHD, these devices often become sources of constant stimulation, making it difficult to concentrate on important tasks.

Identifying this distraction involves recognizing when and how electronic devices interrupt attention. It's like marking the areas where digital paths can take us off course.

2. Noisy Environments: Disconcerting Sounds

Noisy environments are like sound storms that can cloud concentration. Women with ADHD may be especially sensitive to noise, making it difficult to focus on a specific task. Identifying this distraction involves observing how different environments and sounds affect the ability to concentrate.

It's like pointing out the places on the path where noise can become a barrier, preventing you from moving forward clearly.

3. Multiple Tasks: Unstable Balance

Multitasking is like walking on a narrow path. For some women with ADHD, the ability to multitask can be tempting, but it can also lead to a dispersion of attention. Identifying this distraction involves recognizing when multitasking affects the quality of work.

4. Lack of Structure: Roads without Signage

Lack of structure in daily tasks is like navigating unmarked roads. Women with ADHD often find challenges when tasks lack a clear framework. Identifying this distraction involves observing how the lack of structure affects the ability to organize and concentrate.

It would be like pointing out the sections of the road where the absence of signs makes navigation and planning difficult.

5. Wandering Thoughts: Mental Paths

Wandering thoughts are like trails that lead us away from the task at hand. For some women with ADHD, the mind can wander easily, jumping from one thought to another. Identifying this distraction involves being aware of when the mind wanders away from the main task.

How to Identify and Address Common Distractions

Identifying common distractions is the first step to overcoming them. Here are some practical tips:

- **Self-observation :** Taking time to observe and reflect on moments when concentration is affected. This can be done through keeping a diary or log.
- **Solicit Feedback:** Ask friends, family, or colleagues to provide feedback on observed patterns. Often, others can identify distractions that may go unnoticed.
- **Tests and Experimentation:** Carry out small tests and experiments to identify which environments, methods or conditions favor concentration. Learning what works best is essential.
- **Establish Addressing Strategies:** Once distractions are identified, develop specific strategies to address them. This may include creating quieter environments, setting time limits for the use of electronic devices, and breaking down tasks into more manageable steps.
- **Establish Clear Routines:** Creating structured routines can help minimize distractions. This includes allocating specific times for work, rest, and recreational activities.

Benefits of Identifying Common Distractions

Identifying common distractions offers significant benefits for women with ADHD. By recognizing the specific obstacles that impact concentration, the door opens to implement personalized strategies. These approaches not only help overcome distractions, but also encourage greater efficiency and well-being in daily life.

4.2 Techniques to maintain focus

Understanding the Importance of Maintaining Focus

Maintaining focus is like navigating a narrow path; requires constant attention and specific strategies. For women with ADHD, these techniques are key to counteract distractions and move toward their goals. Let's look at some effective techniques to maintain focus:

Task Segmentation: Divide and Conquer

Task segmentation is like dividing the road into manageable sections. Instead of tackling an entire task at once, breaking it down into smaller chunks makes it easier to focus. Women with ADHD are able to approach each segment with greater attention, avoiding the overwhelming feeling that often accompanies extensive tasks.

Pomodoro Techniques : Focus on Blocks of Time

Pomodoro technique is like setting up rest stations along the way. It involves working in specific blocks of time, usually 25 minutes, followed by a short break. This helps maintain concentration by providing defined periods of intense focus, followed by moments of recovery.

Goal Visualization: Images on the Horizon

Goal visualization is like having clear images of the end goal in mind. Women with ADHD may benefit from visualizing the desired outcome before beginning a task. This not only provides motivation, but also helps maintain focus on the purpose of the activity.

Regular Exercise: Renewed Energy on the Road

Regular exercise is like refueling at a gas station. Physical activity not only improves overall health, but also increases energy levels and improves concentration. Women with ADHD can incorporate short exercise breaks throughout the day to stay alert and focused.

Establish Priorities: Clear Signage on the Road

Establishing priorities is like clearly marking the path. By identifying the most important and urgent tasks, women with ADHD can direct their attention to what really matters. This prevents the dispersion of energy on less significant tasks.

Strategic Breaks: Rest Areas on the Trip

Strategic breaks are like planned rest areas on the trip. Taking short breaks between tasks allows women with ADHD to regain energy and maintain mental freshness. These breaks prevent fatigue and contribute to more sustainable performance.

How to Integrate These Techniques into Daily Life

The key to getting the most out of these techniques is to consciously integrate them into daily life. Here are some practical tips:

- **Create Personalized Routines:** Incorporate these techniques into your daily routine consistently. They can be part of the morning, afternoon, or evening, depending on what works best.
- **Adapt to Personal Preferences:** Customize techniques according to individual preferences. What works for one person may not be as effective for another, so it's important to adjust them based on personal needs and styles.
- **Test and Adjust:** Experiment with different combinations and durations of techniques. There is no one-size-fits-all approach, and adjusting techniques based on personal response is essential.
- **Incorporate Gradually:** Introduce these techniques gradually into your daily routine. Sudden changes can be overwhelming, but incorporating the techniques gradually makes adaptation easier.
- **Maintain Consistency:** Consistency is key. Establishing solid habits takes time and consistent practice.

Benefits of Techniques to Maintain Focus

Integrating these techniques into daily life offers significant benefits. By maintaining focus, women with ADHD can experience improvement in efficiency, quality of work, and overall well-being. These techniques not only act as momentary tools, but become constant allies on the path to success and renewed concentration.

4.3 Creation of environments conducive to concentration

Understanding the Influence of the Environment on Concentration

The environment is like the backdrop of our daily lives, and its impact on concentration should not be underestimated. For women with ADHD, certain aspects of the environment can become significant distractions or facilitators that promote attention. Let's see how proper environment configuration can make a difference:

1. Ordered Spaces: Clarity on the Horizon

An orderly space is like a clear path that allows you to move forward without obstacles. For women with ADHD, maintaining an organized, clutter-free environment reduces the chance of visual distractions and makes it easier to focus on the task at hand.

2. Adequate Lighting: Guiding Lights

Proper lighting is like having headlights guiding the way. A well-lit environment helps maintain attention and reduces visual fatigue. Women with ADHD can benefit from balanced lighting that avoids annoying shadows and creates a comfortable environment.

3. Minimize Distracting Noises: Calm on the Road

Reducing distracting noises is like silencing the noise on the road. For women with ADHD, unnecessary sounds can be significant sources of distraction. Setting up a quiet environment, whether by using earplugs or selecting quieter spaces, helps maintain focus.

4. Personalization of Space: Individual Marks on the Path

Customizing space is like leaving individual marks on the road. For women with ADHD, having a space that reflects their personal tastes and needs can improve connection to the task. Decorating the environment with significant elements creates a welcoming and pleasant atmosphere.

5. Eliminate Electronic Distractions: Disconnect to Connect

Eliminating electronic distractions is like turning off the flashing lights on the road. Electronic devices, such as phones and computers, can be major distractions. Setting specific times for use and creating electronics-free zones during certain periods helps maintain focus.

6. Establish Designated Work Zones: Focus Areas

Establishing designated work zones is like marking out specific areas of the road for concentration. Women with ADHD may benefit from allocating specific spaces for particular activities. This creates mental associations that indicate that that place is reserved for tasks that require attention.

How to Set Up Environments Conducive to Concentration

Setting up environments conducive to concentration involves conscious consideration of the elements that impact attention. Here are some practical tips:

- Personalized Observation: Observe how different aspects of the environment affect personal concentration. Each person may have specific preferences, and personalized observation is key to adapting the environment effectively.
- Experiment with Adjustments: Make gradual adjustments to the environment and observe how they affect concentration. Experimenting with different settings allows you to identify what works best.
- Request Feedback: Ask friends, family, or colleagues to provide feedback on the impact of the environment on concentration. Sometimes outside observations can be insightful.
- Create Setup Routines: Establish routines to set up the environment before performing tasks that require concentration. Consistency in settings helps create habits that promote mindfulness.

- Adapt to Task Changes: Adjust the environment according to the specific needs of different tasks. What works for reading may not be best for writing, for example.

Benefits of Creating Environments Conducive to Concentration

Creating environments conducive to concentration offers significant benefits for women with ADHD. By eliminating distractions and setting up spaces that encourage mindfulness, you create an ideal setting for optimal performance. These environments not only act as backdrops, but become constant allies on the journey toward success and renewed focus.

Chapter 5: Personal and Social Relationships

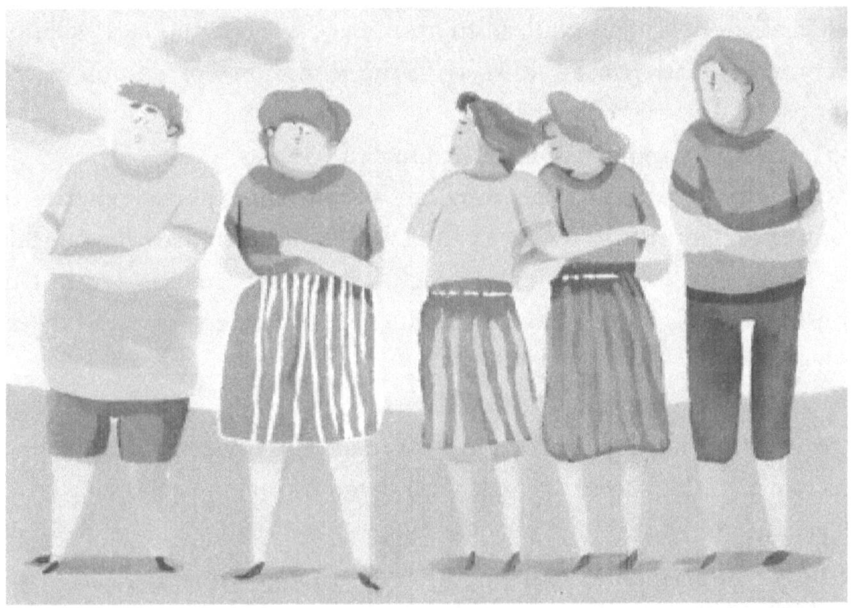

In the complex fabric of life, personal and social relationships represent a fundamental element. For women with Attention Deficit Hyperactivity Disorder (ADHD), these connections can present unique challenges and significant opportunities. In this leg of the journey, we will dive into the impact of ADHD on relationships, exploring how this condition can influence interpersonal dynamics and offering strategies to strengthen emotional bonds. Join us as we unravel the complexity of relationships and discover paths to a deeper, richer connection.

5.1 Impact of ADHD on relationships

Understanding ADHD and Its Effects on Relationships

ADHD is like a unique melody that resonates in the symphony of life. However, this melody can sometimes create unexpected variations in relationship dynamics. Let's look at some key aspects of ADHD's impact on personal connections:

A) Attention and Listening Challenges: The Interrupted Symphony

Scattered attention and difficulty listening can be like discordant notes in communication. For women with ADHD, the ability to pay sustained attention is often challenged, which can lead to misunderstandings and lack of emotional connection in relationships. It is as if the symphony of communication is interrupted by unexpected pauses.

B) Impulsivity in Decisions: Unexpected Chords

Impulsivity in decision making can be like unexpected chords in the harmony of a relationship. Women with ADHD may face challenges in thinking slowly before making decisions, which can affect stability and trust in relationships. It is as if the melody takes unexpected directions, creating tensions in the harmony.

C) Time Management: Uneven Rhythm

Irregular time management can be like an uneven rhythm in the dance of life. Women with ADHD often struggle with organization and following deadlines, which can affect expectations and planning in relationships. It's as if the pace of life varies, creating challenges to stay in sync.

D) Mood Changes: Emotional Nuances

Mood swings can be like emotional nuances in the relationship score. Women with ADHD may experience emotional fluctuations that can affect interpersonal dynamics. It is as if the emotional palette expands, creating vibrant but sometimes unpredictable colors.

E) Hyperfocus : Selective Depth

Hyperfocus can be like a deep dive into a specific note in the relationship . Although there may be a unique ability to focus intensely on certain aspects, this can sometimes lead to a lack of attention on other important elements. It's as if a specific note stands out, but others remain in the background.

<u>Strategies to Strengthen Relationships with ADHD</u>

Despite the challenges, women with ADHD can cultivate strong, nurturing relationships. Here are some strategies to strengthen personal connections:

1. Open and Transparent Communication: Harmonizing the Notes

Encouraging open and transparent communication is like harmonizing the notes of the relationship. Establishing a space where both parties feel comfortable expressing their thoughts and feelings contributes to mutual understanding and conflict resolution. It's like tuning the notes to create a more harmonious melody.

2. Establish Clear Expectations: Setting the Compass

Setting clear expectations is like defining the beat of the relationship. Having open conversations about needs, boundaries, and goals helps create a shared framework. It's like agreeing on the rhythm that best suits both of you in the dance of connection.

3. Develop Joint Routines: Following the Score

Developing joint routines is like following the score of the relationship. Creating shared structures and habits provides stability and predictability in daily dynamics. It's like coordinating movements to maintain synchronization in the dance of life.

4. Practice Empathy: Feeling the Emotional Vibrations

Practicing empathy is like feeling the emotional vibrations of the relationship. Putting yourself in someone else's shoes, understanding their perspectives, and validating their emotions contributes to emotional connection. It's like tuning into emotions to create a deeper resonance.

5. Harness Positive Hyperfocus : Highlighting Special Notes

Taking advantage of the positive hyperfocus is like highlighting the special notes of the relationship. Identifying areas of shared interest and allowing hyperfocus to be directed toward positive aspects strengthens the connection. It's like directing attention to the notes that enrich the melody.

<u>Benefits of Addressing the Impact of ADHD on Relationships</u>

By addressing the impact of ADHD on relationships, women can experience significant benefits. Mutual understanding, strategic adaptation, and building stronger connections contribute to healthier, more satisfying relationships. These efforts not only improve interpersonal dynamics, but also enrich overall quality of life.

5.2 Effective communication with friends and family

Importance of Effective Communication

Effective communication is like a shared language that allows relationships to flourish. For women with ADHD, who may face specific challenges in communication, understanding the importance of conveying thoughts and emotions clearly is essential. Let's look at some key aspects:

Building Mutual Understanding: The Art of Connecting

Effective communication is like a bridge that connects two shores. It allows you to build mutual understanding, where words not only transmit information, but also create emotional connections. For women with ADHD, expressing thoughts and feelings clearly contributes to deeper understanding in relationships.

Resolving Conflicts Constructively: Breaking Down Barriers

Effective communication is like a tool that dismantles barriers. In times of conflict, the ability to express concerns, listen actively, and seek solutions together contributes to resolving challenges constructively. For women with ADHD, addressing conflict with open communication can be key to maintaining healthy relationships.

Strengthening Emotional Bonds: Weaving the Fabric of Connection

Effective communication is like a thread that weaves the fabric of emotional connection. By expressing emotions in an authentic and receptive way, emotional bonds are strengthened. For women with ADHD, who may experience emotional changes, communicating openly and honestly about their feelings contributes to a deeper connection.

Share Goals and Expectations: Navigate Together towards a Common Horizon

Effective communication is like a map that guides you towards common goals. Sharing goals and expectations, discussing plans, and aligning visions contributes to harmony in relationships. For women with ADHD, clarifying expectations through open communication avoids misunderstandings and promotes joint navigation toward the future.

Strategies to Improve Communication with ADHD

Understanding the importance of effective communication is the first step, but it is also essential to have practical strategies to implement in everyday life. Here are some suggestions:

1. Practice Active Listening: Tune the Ears and the Heart

Active listening is like tuning your ears and heart. It involves paying full attention to the person who is speaking, asking questions for clarification, and showing empathy. For women with ADHD, practicing active listening improves mutual understanding and strengthens connections.

2. Use Non-Verbal Communication: Express without Words

Non-verbal communication is like a silent language that complements words. Gestures, facial expressions, and postures can add depth to communication. For women with ADHD, using nonverbal communication helps convey emotions more completely.

3. Establish Conversation Times: Build Dedicated Spaces

Setting specific times to talk is like building dedicated spaces for communication. It can be beneficial to schedule times to discuss important topics, avoiding distractions and allowing full focus on the conversation. For women with ADHD, this makes it easier to concentrate and express clearly.

4. Use Communication Tools: Write, Draw, Record

Communication tools are like extensions of language. Writing, drawing, or keeping a visual record of ideas and feelings can be helpful in expressing thoughts more effectively. For women with ADHD, these tools offer an alternative way to communicate.

5. Set Clear Expectations: Align Personal Maps

Setting clear expectations is like aligning personal maps. Talking openly about expectations and goals in the relationship helps avoid misunderstandings. For women with ADHD, this creates shared ground where both parties understand the direction of the connection.

<u>Benefits of Effective Communication in Relationships with ADHD</u>

Improving communication in relationships with ADHD provides significant benefits. From deeper mutual understanding to constructive conflict resolution, effective communication contributes to stronger, more satisfying relationships. Women with ADHD can experience a more authentic and nurturing connection by implementing strategies that strengthen their ability to express themselves and understand others.

5.3 Building healthy relationships

Understanding Building Healthy Relationships

Building healthy relationships is like the craft of creating strong bridges between people. For women with ADHD, who may face unique challenges in this process, understanding some fundamental principles can be key:

A) Foundations of Trust: The Solid Foundation of Relationships

Trust is like the solid foundation of a building. Building healthy relationships involves establishing a foundation of mutual trust. For women with ADHD, being honest, following through on commitments, and communicating openly helps build this solid foundation.

B) Open Communication: The Bridge of Understanding

Open communication is like the bridge that connects two shores. In building healthy relationships, expressing thoughts and feelings clearly and responsively is essential. For women with ADHD, practicing open communication establishes a channel for mutual understanding.

C) Mutual Respect: Pillars of Reciprocal Support

Mutual respect is like the pillars that support a structure. In healthy relationships, recognizing and valuing individual differences creates a solid foundation. For women with ADHD, understanding and respecting the needs and perspectives of others is essential.

D) Adaptability: Flexibility in Construction

Adaptability is like flexibility in construction. Healthy relationships require the ability to adapt to changes and challenges. For women with ADHD, being open to adjustments and being flexible in relational dynamics contributes to the strength of the connection.

E) Emotional Support: The Support Structure

Emotional support is like the support structure. In healthy relationships, giving and receiving emotional support strengthens the connection. For women with ADHD, recognizing and expressing emotions, as well as offering support to their loved ones, contributes to the strength of the relationship.

Strategies for Building Healthy Relationships with ADHD

Building healthy relationships with ADHD involves specific strategies that align with the characteristics and challenges of this condition. Here are some practical suggestions:

1. Set Clear Expectations

Setting clear expectations is like building the shared framework of the relationship. Having open conversations about goals, limits, and needs helps avoid misunderstandings. For women with ADHD, this clarity contributes to building a strong and understanding relationship.

2. Practice Empathy

Practicing empathy is like recognizing and validating the emotions of another. Putting yourself in your loved one's shoes, understanding their perspectives, and offering emotional support contributes to building a deeper connection. For women with ADHD, empathy is a valuable tool to strengthen the relationship.

3. Develop Positive Habits

Developing positive habits is like sowing seeds of well-being in your relationship. Cultivating gratitude, appreciation, and positive communication contributes to a healthy relational environment. For women with ADHD, incorporating positive habits strengthens emotional connection.

4. Establish Joint Routines

Establishing joint routines is like building routine bridges in the relationship. Creating shared habits provides stability and predictability. For women with ADHD, routines offer structure that contributes to relational strength.

5. Seek External Support

Seeking external support is like strengthening the foundations of the relationship. Engaging in couples therapy or seeking counseling may be beneficial in addressing specific challenges. For women with ADHD, external support offers additional tools and strategies for relationship building.

Benefits of Building Healthy Relationships with ADHD

Building healthy relationships with ADHD not only strengthens personal connections, but also brings significant benefits:

- **Emotional Well-being:** Strong relationships contribute to the emotional well-being of both women with ADHD and their loved ones.

- **Resilience in Challenges:** Relational strength provides a foundation to face challenges and overcome obstacles together.

- **Personal Growth:** Healthy relationships act as supportive spaces for personal growth and individual development.

- **Promoting Authenticity:** A strong relationship allows women with

ADHD to be authentic and feel accepted for who they are.

- **Meaningful Connections:** Building healthy relationships offers deeper, more meaningful connections in life's journey.

Chapter 6: Emotional Management in Women with ADHD

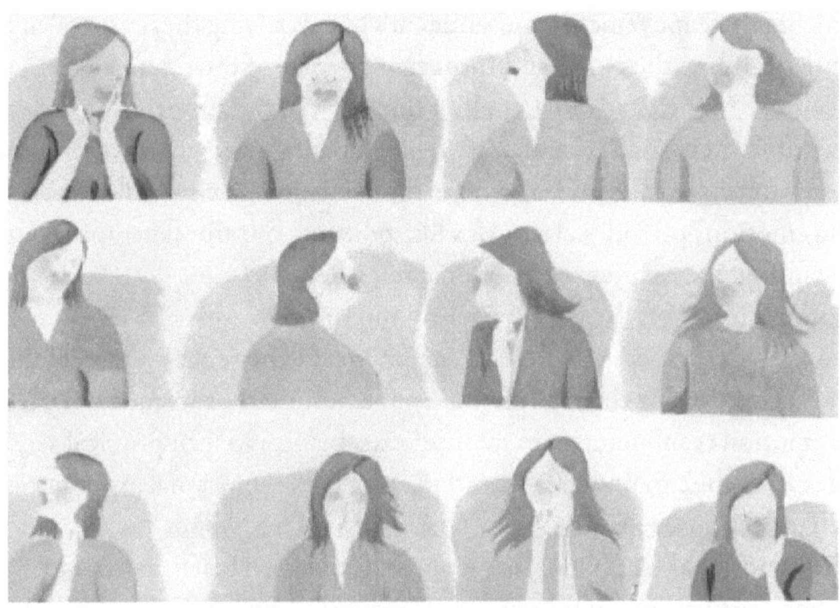

In the vast universe of our experiences, emotions are like stars that illuminate the sky of our existence. For women with Attention Deficit Hyperactivity Disorder (ADHD), understanding and recognizing these emotions can be a fascinating and sometimes challenging journey. On this leg of the journey, we will dive into "Emotion Recognition," exploring how women with ADHD can navigate the changing waters of their feelings with understanding and authenticity. Join us as we unravel strategies that will allow you to recognize and embrace emotions as an integral part of your journey.

6.1 Emotion recognition

The Sea of Emotions: Navigating the Changing Waters

Let's imagine our emotions like waves in an immense and ever-changing sea. For women with ADHD, this sea can present turbulent waters, where emotions can be intense and sometimes difficult to understand. Recognizing these emotions is like learning to navigate, allowing for a safer and more enriching journey. Let's look at some key aspects of emotion recognition:

The Dance of Emotions: Recognizing the Movements

Emotions are like dancers that move on the stage of our mind. For women with ADHD, who may experience more pronounced emotional changes, recognizing these movements is essential. It's like watching the dance of emotions and understanding the twists and turns that are part of the human experience.

Accurate Identification: Labeling the Stars in the Emotional Sky

Identifying emotions accurately is like labeling the stars in the emotional sky. For women with ADHD, whose mind can be a whirlwind of thoughts, naming emotions provides clarity. It's like pointing out the stars in the dark and understanding the richness of emotional nuances.

Connection with the Body: Feeling the Inner Waves

Emotions are intertwined with our physical experiences. Connecting with the body is like feeling the internal waves of emotions. For women with ADHD, whose emotions can manifest in intense ways, being aware of physical sensations provides an avenue to understand and manage these emotional experiences.

Self-Acceptance : Embracing the Emotional Spectrum

The emotional spectrum is wide and diverse. Self -acceptance is like embracing the entire rainbow of emotions. For women with ADHD, recognizing that all emotions are valid and part of the human experience allows for a healthier relationship with their emotional world. It's like accepting all the stars in the sky, without judging their brightness or intensity.

Strategies for the Recognition of Emotions in Women with ADHD

Recognizing emotions is a continuous process that involves practice and authenticity. Here are some practical strategies:

1. Keep an Emotional Diary

Keeping an emotional diary is like mapping your emotions. Recording daily feelings provides clear insight into emotional patterns. For women with ADHD, this offers a valuable tool for understanding and anticipating their emotional responses.

Mindfulness Practice

Mindfulness practice is like anchoring yourself in the present moment. For women with ADHD, who may feel overwhelmed by thoughts and emotions, mindfulness offers a way to focus on the now and acknowledge emotions without judgment.

3. Use of Visual Metaphors

Visual metaphors are like painting the emotional landscape. Creating visual images that represent emotions helps shape and understand internal feelings. For women with ADHD, this offers a concrete way to explore their emotional world.

4. Open Conversations

Open conversations are like sharing the emotional journey with others. Talking about emotions with close friends or loved ones provides outside perspectives and emotional support. For women with ADHD, this strengthens emotional connection and fosters mutual understanding.

5. Integrate Self-Care Practices

Integrating self-care practices is like nurturing the internal garden of emotions. Focusing on activities that promote emotional well-being, such as exercise, meditation or time outdoors, contributes to more balanced emotional management. For women with ADHD, these practices offer essential tools to cultivate their emotional well-being.

Benefits of Emotion Recognition in Women with ADHD

Emotion recognition not only enriches personal understanding, but also provides significant benefits:

- Greater Self-Awareness: Recognizing emotions increases self-awareness, allowing women with ADHD to better understand themselves.
- Better Decision Making: Accurate identification of emotions facilitates informed decision making, contributing to more effective emotional management.
- Strengthening Relationships: The open expression of emotions strengthens emotional connections with others, fostering healthier relationships.
- Stress Reduction: Understanding and recognizing emotions contributes to stress reduction by allowing a more balanced emotional response.
- Promotion of Mental Wellbeing: Emotion recognition is a vital tool to promote mental and emotional well-being on a daily basis.

6.2 Strategies to regulate emotions

<u>Understanding Emotional Regulation</u>

Emotional regulation is like adjusting the volume in an orchestra to achieve harmony. For women with ADHD, whose emotions can be intense and changeable, understanding how to regulate these emotional responses is essential. Let's look at some key strategies:

1. Emotional Mindfulness : Anchoring in the Present

The practice of emotional mindfulness is like anchoring yourself in the present. It involves paying conscious attention to emotions without judging them. For women with ADHD, this offers a valuable tool to manage emotions effectively and reduce emotional reactivity.

2. Conscious Breathing: Calming Emotional Waves

Conscious breathing is like calming emotional waves. By focusing on breathing, emotional intensity can be reduced. For women with ADHD, who may experience emotions more intensely, mindful breathing provides a calming pause.

3. Identifying Emotional Triggers : Dismantling the Underlying Causes

Identifying emotional triggers is like dismantling the underlying causes of emotional responses. For women with ADHD, understanding what situations or events trigger certain emotions is key to addressing them effectively.

4. Regular Self-Care Practices: Nurturing Emotional Well-being

Integrating regular self-care practices is like nurturing emotional well-being. Exercise, healthy eating and adequate rest contribute to lasting emotional balance. For women with ADHD, self-care is essential to staying in tune with their emotions.

5. Creative Expression: Channeling Emotions through Art

Creative expression is like channeling emotions through art. Painting, writing, or engaging in other forms of creative expression allows you to release and explore emotions. For women with ADHD, this offers an avenue to process and understand their feelings.

<u>Practical Strategies to Regulate Emotions in Women with ADHD</u>

Emotional regulation involves practical strategies that adapt to individual needs. Here are some suggestions:

1. Develop Stable Routines: Creating Emotional Anchors. Developing stable routines is like creating emotional anchors. Establishing a daily structure provides predictability, helping women with ADHD feel more confident and in control of their emotions.

2. Visualization Techniques: Imagine the Inner Balance. Visualization techniques are like imagining inner balance. Visualizing a balanced and positive emotional state can influence emotional responses. For women with ADHD, this is a powerful tool to redirect emotions.

3. Establish Personal Boundaries: Protecting Emotional Space. Setting personal boundaries is like protecting emotional space. Deciding when to say no and setting clear limits contributes to more effective emotional regulation. For women with ADHD, this prevents emotional saturation.

4. Practice of Gratitude: Cultivating Emotional Positivity. Practicing gratitude is like cultivating emotional positivity. Focusing on positive aspects of life helps counteract negative emotions. For women with ADHD, gratitude is a tool that promotes emotional well-being.

5. Psychological Therapy: Exploring Personalized Strategies. Psychological therapy is like exploring personalized strategies. Working with a professional can provide specific tools to regulate emotions and address unique emotional challenges. For women with ADHD, this offers a space for support and learning.

<u>Benefits of Emotional Regulation in Women with ADHD</u>

Emotional regulation not only contributes to individual well-being, but also provides significant benefits:

- **Stress Reduction:** Emotional regulation reduces stress by offering tools to manage intense emotional responses.
- **Better Decision Making:** Managing emotions allows for more informed and balanced decision making.
- **Strengthening Relationships:** Emotional regulation contributes to healthier relationships by avoiding impulsive reactions.
- **Mental Wellbeing:** Emotional regulation is essential for mental well-being, allowing women with ADHD to deal with emotional challenges effectively.
- **Development of Resilience :** The ability to regulate emotions

promotes resilience , allowing us to overcome adversities with greater strength.

6.3 Impact of ADHD on mental health and emotional well-being

Understanding the Emotional Terrain of ADHD

ADHD is like a unique emotional landscape, where mountains of distraction and currents of hyperactivity can affect internal balance. Let's see how this specific terrain can influence mental health and emotional well-being:

A) Emotional Intensity: Waves That Can Break Strong

Women with ADHD may experience a unique emotional intensity. It's like having emotional waves that can break hard on the beach of your lives. This intensity can affect the way emotions are processed and managed, adding challenges to the emotional journey.

B) Challenges in Attention and Concentration: Navigating Fast Currents

The fast currents of ADHD can make it difficult to focus and concentrate. It's like navigating turbulent waters where staying emotionally on track can be a challenge. Constant distraction can impact the ability to focus on emotions and fully understand them.

ADHD can also influence self-esteem and lead to self-criticism. It's like walking on rocky trails where inner thoughts can be more challenging. Women with ADHD may face moments of self-doubt and internal criticism that affect their perception of themselves.

D) Coping Strategies: Building Resilient Bridges

Despite the challenges, it is essential to note that women with ADHD also develop unique coping strategies. It's like building resilient bridges over emotional rivers. By understanding and addressing these challenges, women with ADHD can cultivate tools that strengthen their emotional well-being.

Impact of ADHD on Mental Health and Emotional Well-being

1. Anxiety and Stress. ADHD can contribute to higher levels of anxiety and stress. Difficulties in attention and concentration can lead to constant worries, contributing to anxiety. It is important to recognize and address these aspects to reduce the impact on mental health.

2. Depression and Discouragement. The constant struggle with attention and task management can lead to feelings of discouragement and, in some cases, depression. It's like walking down a steep path where your mood can be affected. Identifying these feelings and seeking support is crucial to addressing mental health.

3. Challenges in Personal Relationships. ADHD can impact personal relationships. Difficulties in attention can affect communication and emotional connection. Navigating these waters requires patience and understanding from those around women with ADHD.

4. Self-esteem and Self-concept . Self-esteem and self-concept can be affected by the challenges associated with ADHD. It is important to recognize personal achievements and strengths, building a positive image of themselves. Self-compassion and acceptance are powerful tools in this process.

Strategies to Improve Mental Health and Emotional Well-being in Women with ADHD

- Psychological Therapy: Exploring Personalized Strategies. Psychological therapy is like exploring personalized strategies to address the specific challenges of ADHD. Working with a professional offers a supportive and learning space to manage anxiety, depression and other aspects of mental health.

- Social Support: Building Support Networks. Social support is like building strong support networks. Maintaining healthy connections with friends and family offers invaluable support. Open communication about ADHD and its challenges can strengthen these relationships.

- Self-Care Practices: Nurturing General Well-being. Self-care practices are like nurturing overall well-being. Incorporating activities that promote emotional balance, such as exercise, meditation, and time outdoors, contributes to emotional well-being.

- Education and Awareness: Understanding and Communicating ADHD. Education and awareness are how to understand and communicate ADHD. Educating yourself about the condition and sharing this information with friends, family and colleagues helps create an environment of understanding and support.

Benefits of Mental Health Care and Emotional Well-being in Women with ADHD

Attention to mental health and emotional well-being not only improves the quality of life of women with ADHD, but also provides significant benefits:

- **Stress Reduction:** Addressing mental health reduces stress and contributes to a more balanced emotional response.
- **Improvement in Personal Relationships:** Working on emotional well-being strengthens personal relationships by promoting communication and mutual understanding.
- **Resilience Development :** Addressing emotional challenges promotes resilience , allowing you to face adversity with greater strength.
- **Promotion of Self-Awareness:** Addressing mental health facilitates self-knowledge, allowing women with ADHD to better understand themselves and develop effective strategies.
- **Contribution to Personal Success:** Attention to mental health and emotional well-being are fundamental pillars for personal success and the achievement of long-term goals.

Chapter 7: Financial Control and ADHD

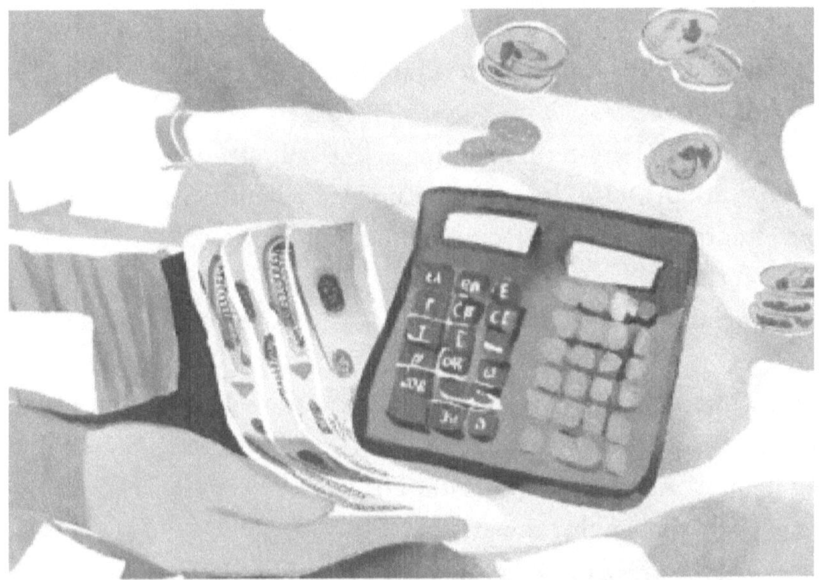

In the vast terrain of everyday life, finances are like a river that flows through our days, affecting every aspect of our existence. For women with Attention Deficit Hyperactivity Disorder (ADHD), this river can present unique challenges that impact their ability to navigate the financial waters fluidly. In this leg of the journey, we will explore the "Financial Challenges Associated with ADHD", unraveling the complexities that arise in money management and providing practical strategies to overcome these obstacles.

7.1 Financial challenges associated with ADHD

1. Distractions and Disorganization: A Welter of Invoices and Documents

Distraction and disorganization, central characteristics of ADHD, can turn managing invoices and financial documents into a tidal wave. It's like trying to stay on course on a ship while waves of papers pile up. This challenge can lead to late payments, financial forgetfulness, and frustration.

2. Financial Impulsiveness: Strong Winds in Spending Decisions

Impulsivity, another facet of ADHD, can manifest itself in quick and sometimes poorly thought-out financial decisions. It's like sailing in waters where the winds of impulsiveness can change the direction of the financial ship without warning. This tendency can contribute to unnecessary spending and a lack of long-term planning.

3. Difficulties in Long-Term Planning: Navigating without a Clear Course

The difficulty in long-term planning is like sailing without a clear direction. For women with ADHD, long-term vision may be obscured by challenges in sustained attention. This can affect the ability to set long-term financial goals and save for the future.

4. Financial Stress and Anxiety: Emotional Storms on the Financial Horizon

Financial stress and anxiety can be like emotional storms on the financial horizon. Constant worries about money can increase emotional burden, affecting mental and emotional health. For women with ADHD, these storms can be especially challenging to navigate.

<u>Practical Strategies to Overcome Financial Challenges with ADHD</u>

A) Establishing Financial Routines: Anchors in a Sea of Challenges

Establishing financial routines is like creating anchors in a sea of challenges. Scheduling specific times to review bills, budget, and organize documents helps maintain financial stability. For women with ADHD, these routines act as reference points amidst distractions.

B) Use of Technological Tools: Digital Compasses in the Financial World

The use of technological tools is like having digital compasses in the financial world. Apps and programs designed for financial management can be valuable allies for women with ADHD. Automating payments and setting reminders helps avoid forgetfulness and delays.

C) Establish Realistic Financial Goals: Navigate Toward Achievable Horizons

Setting realistic financial goals is like navigating toward achievable horizons. For women with ADHD, it is crucial to set goals that are specific and achievable. This facilitates short- and long-term planning, reducing anxiety associated with financial uncertainty.

D) Consult with Financial Professionals: Captains in Uncharted Waters

Consulting with financial professionals is like having expert captains in uncharted waters. Seeking expert advice can provide clarity and direction. Financial advisors can help establish personalized strategies that fit specific needs and challenges.

E) Incorporate Reflective Pauses: Avoid the Winds of Impulsivity

Incorporating reflective pauses is like avoiding the winds of impulsiveness. Before making important financial decisions, taking a moment to reflect helps reduce the likelihood of impulsive spending. For women with ADHD, this pause offers space to evaluate long-term consequences.

7.2 Tools for financial management

<u>Navigating Financial Tools Adapted to ADHD</u>

Let's imagine that managing finances is like navigating a vast and changing ocean. For women with ADHD, using specific tools can make this journey more manageable. Some key tools include:

1. Budget Apps: Compasses in the Financial World

Budgeting apps are like compasses in the financial world. These tools, like Mint or YNAB (You Need A Budget), allow you to track income and expenses in a clear and organized way. For women with ADHD, these apps offer a visual view of their finances, making it easier to make informed decisions.

2. Automated Alerts and Reminders: Lighthouses on the Financial Horizon

Automated alerts and reminders are like beacons on the financial horizon. Setting automatic reminders for bill payments and other financial tasks prevents forgetfulness and delays. For women with ADHD, these alerts serve as guides to help stay on track amid distractions.

3. Online Banking: Navigating Through Transactions with Ease

Online banking is like navigating through transactions with ease. Accessing bank accounts and making transactions from the comfort of home simplifies daily financial management. For women with ADHD, this accessibility reduces the burden associated with in-person financial tasks.

4. Automatic Savings Apps: Building Reserves Effortlessly

Automatic savings apps are like effortless booking builders. Tools like Digit or Acorns allow you to automatically save small amounts of money. For women with ADHD, this strategy helps build savings gradually, without the need for constant effort.

5. Expense Tracking Tools: Detailed Financial Spending Maps

Expense tracking tools are like detailed maps of financial spending. Apps like PocketGuard or Expensify provide a clear view of how money is spent. For women with ADHD, this visibility makes it easier to identify spending patterns and make informed decisions.

6. Virtual Financial Advisors: Captains in Financial Navigation

Virtual financial advisors are like captains in financial navigation. Platforms like Betterment or Wealthfront offer automated financial advice. For women with ADHD, this option provides professional guidance without the need for in-person appointments, simplifying the financial planning process.

How These Tools Benefit Women with ADHD

A) They Simplify Daily Financial Management :

Budgeting, push alerts, and online banking apps simplify daily financial management. For women with ADHD, this simplification reduces the cognitive load associated with everyday financial tasks.

B) They Offer Visibility and Control:

Expense tracking tools and automatic savings apps offer visibility and control over finances. This is especially beneficial for women with ADHD, allowing them to make informed decisions and follow a clearer financial path.

C) They Facilitate Automatic Savings:

Automatic savings apps make it easy to build savings without constant effort. For women with ADHD, this automation eliminates the need to remember and perform manual actions, encouraging the habit of saving.

D) They Provide Professional Financial Guidance:

Virtual financial advisors offer professional guidance without the need for in-person appointments. For women with ADHD, this removes barriers and provides access to specialized financial advice in a more accessible way.

E) Reduce Financial Stress:

Together, these tools work to reduce financial stress. Clarity, automation, and accessibility simplify money management, contributing to the emotional and financial well-being of women with ADHD.

7.3 Long-term planning and financial goals

Navigating into the Future: The Importance of Long-Term Planning

Let's imagine long-term planning as the act of charting a path toward the future, a future that we want and that reflects our aspirations. For women with ADHD, this process can present unique challenges, but it also offers opportunities to cultivate a long-term sense of direction and achievement. Some key elements of long-term planning include:

<u>Goal Visualization: Painting the Picture of the Desired Future</u>

Visualizing goals is like painting the picture of your desired future. Before embarking on any trip, it is essential to have a clear idea of where you want to go. For women with ADHD, visualizing financial goals provides a visual guide that acts as motivation.

<u>Setting Realistic Goals: Setting Achievable Milestones</u>

Setting realistic goals is like marking achievable milestones on the map. Goals should be specific, measurable and attainable. For women with ADHD, setting realistic goals reduces feelings of overwhelm and facilitates gradual progress.

<u>Developing an Action Plan: Working with a Detailed Map</u>

Developing an action plan is like working with a detailed map. This plan includes specific steps to achieve each goal. For women with ADHD, having a clear plan provides a structure that makes it easier to organize and follow through.

<u>Incorporating Flexibility: Adapting to Changes in Course</u>

Incorporating flexibility is like adapting to changes in direction. On the financial journey, unforeseen events can arise. For women with ADHD, the ability to adjust course without losing sight of long-term goals is key to overcoming unexpected challenges.

<u>Celebrating Intermediate Accomplishments: Recognizing Progress</u>

Celebrating intermediate achievements is like recognizing progress on the journey. Every milestone reached deserves to be celebrated, providing additional motivation. For women with ADHD, this practice fosters a sense of accomplishment and reinforces the connection between effort and reward.

Strategies to Set and Achieve Financial Goals with ADHD

1. Identify Clear and Specific Goals: Before embarking on long-term planning, it is essential to identify clear and specific goals. Is it buying a house, paying off debt, or saving for education? Defining goals provides direction and purpose.

2. Prioritize Goals by Importance : Once the goals are identified, it is crucial to prioritize them by importance. This helps concentrate energy on the most significant objectives and avoids the dispersion of efforts.

3. Break Goals into Small Steps: Breaking goals into small steps makes planning and tracking easier. For women with ADHD, tackling tasks in manageable chunks reduces feelings of overwhelm and facilitates consistent progress.

4. Use Visual Reminders: Visual reminders are powerful tools for women with ADHD. Placing visual goal reminders in visible locations acts as a constant stimulus, keeping goals at the center of attention.

5. Set Realistic Deadlines: Setting realistic deadlines provides a time frame for achieving goals. It is essential to be realistic when assigning deadlines, allowing flexibility without compromising urgency.

6. Seek Support and Accountability: Sharing goals with friends, family or mentors provides support and accountability. Having a support system helps maintain focus and offers valuable perspectives.

How Setting and Achieving Financial Goals Benefits Women with ADHD

Encourages Organization and Focus: Setting and achieving financial goals encourages organization and focus. For women with ADHD, having a clear purpose provides a structure that makes it easier to focus.

Promotes Motivation and Sense of Achievement: Achieving financial goals promotes motivation and a sense of accomplishment. Celebrating each milestone achieved reinforces the connection between effort and reward, boosting self-esteem.

Generates Clarity in Financial Decisions: Long-term planning generates clarity in financial decisions. Having defined goals facilitates making informed decisions and reduces impulsivity.

Contributes to Financial and Emotional Well-being: Setting and achieving financial goals contributes to financial and emotional well-being. For women with ADHD, this means building a solid foundation for the future and reducing anxiety associated with financial uncertainty.

Conclusion

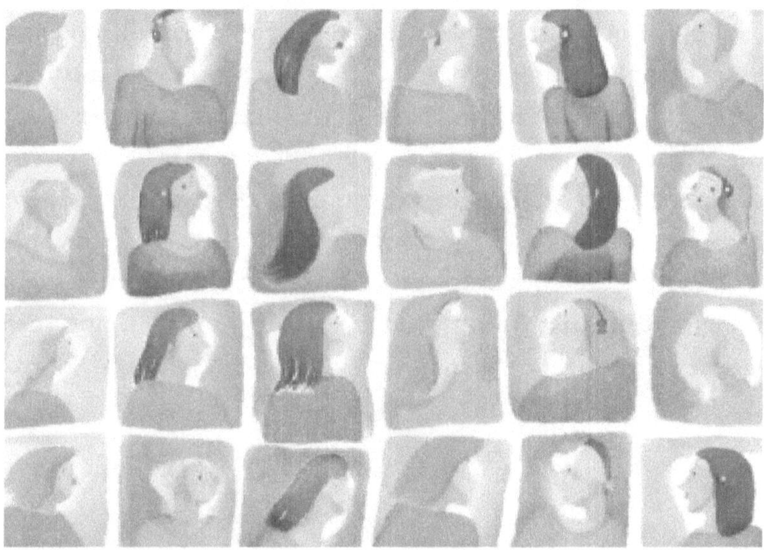

This book has been more than a compendium of tools; has been a beacon of light, guiding us through the unique challenges women with ADHD face and providing a clear map to success in life.

We have explored the complexities of attention and hyperactivity, unraveling gender differences and addressing the specific challenges faced by women with ADHD. Along the way, we've learned about the diagnosis process, breaking down common obstacles, and discovering specialized tools that offer clarity on the path to understanding and self-care.

Organization and time management have been fundamental pillars in our journey, where we have developed skills, created effective routines and explored the power of technological tools to win the battle against everyday distractions. In our personal and social relationships, we have examined the impact of ADHD, learning to communicate effectively and building healthy relationships that enrich our lives.

In the emotional field, we have explored the depth of our emotions, discovering strategies to recognize them, regulate them and maintain lasting emotional balance. We have left no corner unexplored, and we have understood how ADHD intertwines with our finances, unraveling challenges and building bridges to financial control and financial security.

Each chapter has been an adventure, each word a compass that has guided us towards authenticity, understanding and personal growth. We have approached each topic with the belief that while ADHD can present challenges, it also offers opportunities to develop unique skills, cultivate resilience, and succeed in life.

As we close this book, let us remember that the journey does not end here; rather, this is the beginning of an ongoing path toward empowerment and self-actualization. Every strategy, every piece of advice and every story shared has been a link in the chain of our own evolution. Let us continue to navigate together, supporting each other on the journey, and always remember that, with determination and the right tools, women with ADHD can not only succeed, but also shine with their own light in the world. Go ahead, brave ADHD navigators, success awaits you!

Did you love *Women with ADHD*? Then you should read *Amor con ansiedad: Cómo construir relaciones saludables en tiempos inciertos*[1] by Olivia I. Thigpen (ESP)!

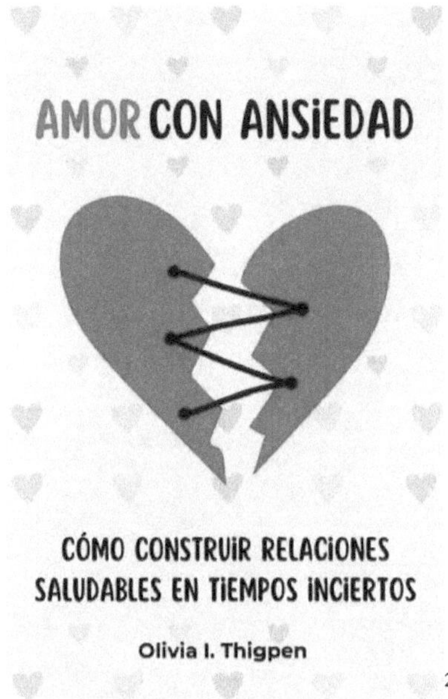

[2]

¡Descubre el camino hacia relaciones más fuertes y amorosas en medio de la ansiedad y la incertidumbre! "Amor con Ansiedad: Cómo Construir Relaciones Saludables en Tiempos Inciertos" es tu guía comprensiva para transformar los desafíos emocionales en oportunidades de crecimiento y conexión genuina.

Este libro te lleva de la mano a través de las complejidades del amor en situaciones difíciles. Explora los diferentes tipos de ansiedad que pueden afectar tus relaciones y aprende a reconocer los síntomas antes de que se conviertan en obstáculos insuperables. Descubre las causas subyacentes de la ansiedad en el contexto de las relaciones de pareja y cómo estas preocupaciones pueden fortalecer, en lugar de debilitar, tu vínculo.

---

1. https://books2read.com/u/3kBlxN

2. https://books2read.com/u/3kBlxN

Dentro de estas páginas, encontrarás estrategias prácticas y científicamente respaldadas para manejar la ansiedad tanto individualmente como en pareja. Aprende a comunicarte de manera efectiva, incluso cuando la ansiedad amenaza con distorsionar tus palabras. Descubre cómo mantener la intimidad y fomentar conexiones más profundas, incluso en los momentos más desafiantes.

Además, enfrenta la incertidumbre con valentía y aprende a convertirla en una oportunidad para fortalecer tu relación. Este libro no solo te proporciona herramientas prácticas para afrontar los desafíos de la vida, sino que también te brinda un enfoque compasivo y esperanzador para enfrentar la ansiedad y la incertidumbre junto a tu ser querido.

"Amor con Ansiedad" no es solo un libro; es una brújula emocional que te guiará a través de las tormentas hacia aguas más serenas y amorosas. Escrito con empatía y respaldado por la ciencia, este libro te empoderará para transformar la ansiedad en un motor de crecimiento personal y amor duradero.

¡Descubre cómo el amor puede florecer incluso en los momentos más oscuros!

Read more at https://oliviatda.com/.

Also by Olivia I. Thigpen ENG

Healthy Mind

The Overthinking Cure: 8 Proven Strategies to Free Your Mind from Negative Spirals, Reduce Stress, Boost Productivity, and Live in the Present Moment
Love amidst Anxiety: How to Build Healthy Relationships in Uncertain Times
Women with ADHD

Healthy Relationships

Breaking Free from Narcissistic Manipulation: Strategies for Healing and Thriving Beyond Toxic Relationships
Narcissistic Relationships: Overcoming Codependency, Setting Boundaries, and Healing Romantic Bonds in a Turbulent World

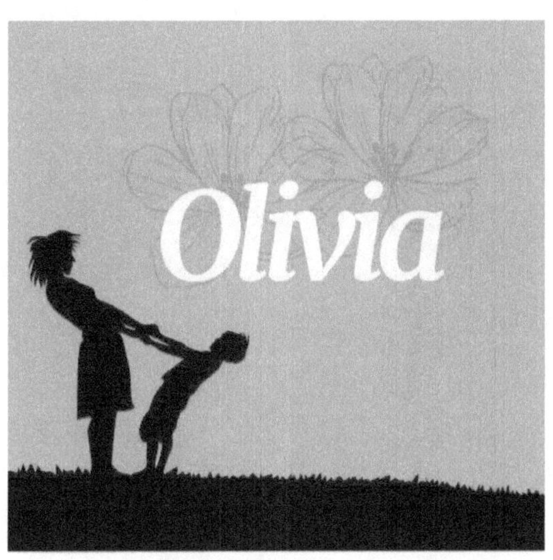

About the Author

Olivia I. Thigpen is a frenetic, multitasking woman. She began her career as an elementary school teacher, but her passion for psychology led her down a different path. She decided to pursue a bachelor's degree in psychology and it wasn't long before she became a psychiatrist. Her experience in her field gave her a wealth of knowledge that would later prove invaluable to her in her career as a writer.